This report contains the collective views of an international group of experts and does not necessarily represent the decisions or the stated policy of the United Nations Environment Programme, the International Labour Organisation, or the World Health Organization

Environmental Health Criteria 42

TECNAZENE

Published under the joint sponsorship of
the United Nations Environment Programme,
the International Labour Organisation,
and the World Health Organization

World Health Organization
Geneva, 1984

The **International Programme on Chemical Safety (IPCS)** is a joint venture of the United Nations Environment Programme, the International Labour Organisation, and the World Health Organization. The main objective of the IPCS is to carry out and disseminate evaluations of the effects of chemicals on human health and the quality of the environment. Supporting activities include the development of epidemiological, experimental laboratory, and risk-assessment methods that could produce internationally comparable results, and the development of manpower in the field of toxicology. Other activities carried out by IPCS include the development of know-how for coping with chemical accidents, coordination of laboratory testing and epidemiological studies, and promotion of research on the mechanisms of the biological action of chemicals.

ISBN 92 4 154182 2

PRINTED IN FINLAND

84/6232 – VAMMALA – 5500

CONTENTS

Page

TASK GROUP MEETING ON ENVIRONMENTAL HEALTH CRITERIA FOR ORGANOCHLORINE PESTICIDES OTHER THAN DDT (ENDOSULFAN, QUINTOZENE, TECNAZENE, TETRADIFON)

Members

Dr E. Astolfi, Faculty of Medicine of Buenos Aires, Buenos Aires, Argentina

Dr I. Desi, Department of Environmental Hygienic Toxicology, National Institute of Hygiene, Budapest, Hungary

Dr R. Drew, Department of Clinical Pharmacology, Flinders University of South Australia, Bedford Park, South Australia

Dr S.K. Kashyap, National Institute of Occupational Health, Ahmedabad, India

Dr A.N. Mohammed, University of Calabar, Calabar, Nigeria

Dr O.E. Paynter, Office of Pesticide Programs, US Environmental Protection Agency, Washington DC, USA

Dr W.O. Phoon, Department of Social Medicine and Public Health, Faculty of Medicine, University of Singapore, Outram Hill, Singapore (Chairman)

Dr D. Wassermann, Department of Occupational Health, The Hebrew University, Hadassah Medical School, Jerusalem, Israel

Representatives of Other Organizations

Dr H. Kaufmann, International Group of National Associations of Agrochemical Manufacturers (GIFAP)

Dr V.E.F. Solman, International Union for Conservation of Nature and Natural Resources (IUCN), Ottawa, Ontario, Canada

Secretariat

Dr S. Dobson, Institute of Terrestrial Ecology, Monks Wood Experimental Station, Abbots Ripton, Huntingdon, United Kingdom (Temporary Adviser)

Secretariat (contd).

Dr M. Gilbert, International Register for Potentially Toxic Chemicals, United Nations Environment Programme, Geneva, Switzerland

Dr K.W. Jager, Division of Environmental Health, International Programme on Chemical Safety, World Health Organization, Geneva, Switzerland (Secretary)

Dr D.C. Villeneuve, Health Protection Branch, Department of National Health and Welfare, Tunney's Pasture, Ottawa, Ontario, Canada (Temporary Adviser) (Rapporteur)

Mr J.D. Wilbourn, Unit of Carcinogen Identification and Evaluation, International Agency for Research on Cancer, Lyons, France

NOTE TO READERS OF THE CRITERIA DOCUMENTS

While every effort has been made to present information in the criteria documents as accurately as possible without unduly delaying their publication, mistakes might have occurred and are likely to occur in the future. In the interest of all users of the environmental health criteria documents, readers are kindly requested to communicate any errors found to the Manager of the International Programme on Chemical Safety, World Health Organization, Geneva, Switzerland, in order that they may be included in corrigenda, which will appear in subsequent volumes.

In addition, experts in any particular field dealt with in the criteria documents are kindly requested to make available to the WHO Secretariat any important published information that may have inadvertently been omitted and which may change the evaluation of health risks from exposure to the environmental agent under examination, so that the information may be considered in the event of updating and re-evaluation of the conclusions contained in the criteria documents.

* * *

A detailed data profile and a legal file can be obtained from the International Register of Potentially Toxic Chemicals, Palais des Nations, 1211 Geneva 10, Switzerland (Telephone no. 988400 - 985850).

ENVIRONMENTAL HEALTH CRITERIA FOR TECNAZENE

Following the recommendations of the United Nations Conference on the Human Environment held in Stockholm in 1972, and in response to a number of World Health Resolutions (WHA23.60, WHA24.47, WHA25.58, WHA26.68), and the recommendation of the Governing Council of the United Nations Environment Programme, (UNEP/GC/10, 3 July 1973), a programme on the integrated assessment of the health effects of environmental pollution was initiated in 1973. The programme, known as the WHO Environmental Health Criteria Programme, has been implemented with the support of the Environment Fund of the United Nations Environment Programme. In 1980, the Environmental Health Criteria Programme was incorporated into the International Programme on Chemical Safety (IPCS). The result of the Environmental Health Criteria Programme is a series of criteria documents.

A WHO Task Group on Environmental Health Criteria for Organochlorine Pesticides other than DDT (Endosulfan, Quintozene, Tecnazene, Tetradifon) was held at the Health Protection Branch, Department of National Health and Welfare Ottawa from 28 May - 1 June, 1984. The meeting was opened by Dr E. Somers, Director- General, Environmental Health Directorate, and Dr K.W. Jager welcomed the participants on behalf of the three co-sponsoring organizations of the IPCS (UNEP/ILO/WHO). The Task Group reviewed and revised the draft criteria document and made an evaluation of the health risks of exposure to tecnazene.

The drafts of this document were prepared by Dr D.C. Villeneuve of Canada and Dr S. Dobson of the United Kingdom.

The efforts of all who helped in the preparation and finalization of the document are gratefully acknowledged.

* * *

Partial financial support for the publication of this criteria document was kindly provided by the United States Department of Health and Human Services, through a contract from the National Institute of Environmental Health Sciences, Research Triangle Park, North Carolina, USA - a WHO Collaborating Centre for Environmental Health Effects.

1. SUMMARY AND RECOMMENDATIONS

1.1 Summary

1.1.1 Identity, analytical methods and sources of exposure

Technical tecnazene (2,3,5,6-tetrachloronitrobenzene), is an odourless, crystalline solid that is used in its formulated form as a fungicide and as a sprout inhibitor on stored potatoes. Gas chromatography with electron capture detection is the preferred method for its determination.

Exposure of the general population is expected to be mainly through residues in food. The residues reported are below the FAO/WHO maximum residue levels.

No cases of accidental or occupational overexposure have been reported.

1.1.2 Environmental concentrations and exposures

Tecnazene is rapidly lost from treated soil, probably mainly through evaporation.

1.1.3 Kinetics and metabolism

Tecnazene is rapidly absorbed and metabolized in the rat and the rabbit following oral administration. High single oral doses (3000 mg in rabbit) are predominantly passed unchanged in the faeces. Several metabolities are presumed in urine, the most important being the mercapturic acid conjugate.

1.1.4 Studies on experimental animals

Tecnazene is only slightly toxic according to the scale of Hodge & Sterner (1956). The oral LD_{50} of tecnazene in the rat is 7500 mg/kg body weight. WHO (1984) has classified tecnazene in the category of technical products unlikely to present an acute hazard in normal use.

In long-term studies, no-observed-adverse-effect levels were:

rat: 750 mg/kg diet for 104 weeks, equivalent to 38 mg/kg body weight per day;

mouse: 1500 mg/kg diet, equivalent to 200 mg/kg body weight per day; and

dog: 15 mg/kg body weight per day (administered orally by capsule for 2 years).

At higher dosages (4000 mg/kg in diets with rats and 240 mg/kg body weight in dogs), growth inhibition occurs and in dogs, the plasma alkaline phosphatase levels increase.

In the tests conducted so far, tecnazene did not affect reproduction (rats), nor was it embryotoxic or teratogenic (rats and mice). No information on mutagenicity and other related short-term tests is available. Data available from a mouse and a rat study do not indicate that tecnazene is a carcinogen.

1.1.5 Effects on man

Dermal sensitivity has been reported in agricultural workers.

1.1.6 Effects on the environment

A lack of effect on bacteria of the nitrogen cycle has been reported, but no other relevant information has been found.

1.2 Recommendations

1. Monitoring studies on occupationally-exposed workers, especially workers in greenhouses, are required concerning both levels of exposure and potential health effects.

2. More data should be made available on tecnazene levels in greenhouse crops.

3. The dermal toxicity, skin sensitization, and eye irritation capacity of tecnazene should be determined in both experimental animals and in the occupational setting.

4. The genotoxicity and cell transformation capacity of tecnazene should be studied. If these studies indicate a need for it, an adequate carcinogenicity study should be done.

5. The level of hexachlorobenzene as an impurity in tecnazene should be kept as low as possible.

2. IDENTITY, PROPERTIES AND ANALYTICAL METHODS

2.1 Identity

Chemical structure:

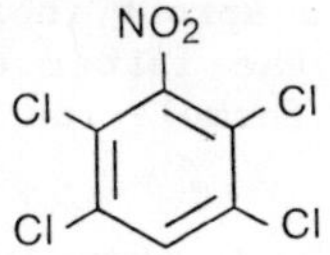

Molecular formula: $C_6HCl_4NO_2$

CAS chemical name: 2,3,5,6-tetrachloronitrobenzene

Common trade names: Chipman 3,142, Folosan, Fusarex, Fumite, Folosan DB905, TCNB

CAS registry Number: 117-18-0

Relative molecular mass: 260.88

2.2 Properties and Analytical Methods

2.2.1 Physical and chemical properties

Tecnazene is a colourless, odourless, crystalline solid with a melting point of 99 °C. It is fairly volatile at room temperature. It is readily soluble in carbon disulfide, benzene, chloroform, ketones, and aromatic and chlorinated hydrocarbon compounds. It is practically insoluble in water (0.44 mg/litre at 20 °C), and its solubility in ethanol is 40 g/litre at 25 °C (Worthing, 1979). Tecnazene is generally very stable; it can be dispersed by pyrotechnic mixtures. It decomposes slowly in solution when exposed to ultraviolet radiation. The technical grade material is more than 99% pure and contains less than 1% of hexachlorobenzene.

2.2.2 Analytical methods

Polarographic, colorimetric, and gas chromatography combined with a flame detector method are described in the literature, but gas chromatography with an electron-capture detector is the preferred method for the determination of tecnazene residues (Dalziel & Duncan, 1974; FAO/WHO, 1979). The limit of detection with this method is approximately 0.01 mg/kg with a recovery of more than 90% (FAO/WHO, 1979).

3. USES, ENVIRONMENTAL LEVELS AND EXPOSURES, TRANSPORT AND DISTRIBUTION

3.1 Uses

Tecnazene is used as a sprout inhibitor on stored potatoes and as a fungicide. In the latter application it is mainly used as a smoke generator formulation in greenhouses (Table 1).

Table 1. Usage data for tecnazene in selected countries[a]

Area	Quantity	Year	Use
Sweden	200 kg	1981	horticultural use against fungi in greenhouses
United Kingdom	0.14 tonne per year	1975-79	fungicide and sprout suppressant; used as a dust or spray on potatoes in storage
USA	unknown	1981	fungicide

[a] From: IRPTC, personal communication, 1984.

3.2 Environmental Levels and Exposures

No data are available on levels in air and water, or on occupational exposure levels.

3.2.1 Levels in food

Washing, peeling, and cooking potatoes reduced levels of tecnazene (Dalziel & Duncan, 1974). Potatoes that had been treated with 3% tecnazene at a rate of 4.5 g/kg were found to contain 3 mg/kg, after 4 - 5 months storage (FAO/WHO, 1979). Washing reduced the levels of tecnazene to below 1 mg/kg, and peeling further reduced the levels to below 0.1 mg/kg. Another 50% loss of tecnazene occured when the peeled potatoes were boiled. Market basket surveys in the USA of about 300 potato samples revealed that 14 samples had detectable residues of tecnazene (i.e., 0.001 mg/kg or more). Trace levels (0.01 mg/kg or less) of tecnazene were found in 15 out of 3500 samples of USA foodstuffs (FAO/WHO, 1979). Analyses of vegetable products in Belgium and Sweden for tecnazene revealed that most of the lettuce, chicory, mushrooms, carrots, sweet peppers, corn, etc., had levels between 0.001 and 0.01 mg/kg fresh weight (Valange, 1974; FAO/WHO, 1979).

The WHO/FAO (1979) has recommended temporary maximum residue (tolerance) levels (MRL) for tecnazene (Table 2).

Table 2. Temporary maximum residue (tolerance) levels (MRL) for tecnazene

Commodity	Temporary MRL (mg/kg)
Lettuce	2
Potatoes (washed before analysis)	1
Chicory (witloot)	0.2
Other vegetables	0.1
Tomatoes	0.1

3.2.2 General population exposure

Environmental exposure is probably low due to its limited use outdoors.

3.3 Transport and Distribution

Tecnazene is rapidly lost from sandy soil, probably mainly because of its volatility (FAO/WHO, 1979).

4. KINETICS AND METABOLISM

Rabbits receiving a single oral dose of 0.1 - 3.0 g/animal eliminated 60 - 78% in the faeces within 3 days, while the urine accounted for 35 - 38% (primarily as conjugated products). At 0.01 g/animal, 22 - 30% was recovered in the faeces (Bray et al., 1953).

Mercapturic acid conjugate was excreted at a rate of 11% within 48 h of the administration of 1 - 3 g of tecnazene to rabbits. Other metabolites excreted included an ether glucuronide (12%), 2,3,5,6-tetrachloroaniline (10%), unconjugated 4-amine-2,3,5,6-tetrachlorophenol (2%) and an etheral sulfate (1%) (Bray et al., 1953; Betts et al., 1955). A suggested pathway for the biotransformation of tecnazene in rabbits based on data obtained from Betts et al. (1955) is shown in Fig. 1. Similar amounts of mercapturic acid were excreted in the urine of rats dosed with tecnazene (Barnes et al., 1959). Tecnazene administered orally to pigeons was converted to mercapturic acid (Wit & Reenwangh, 1969).

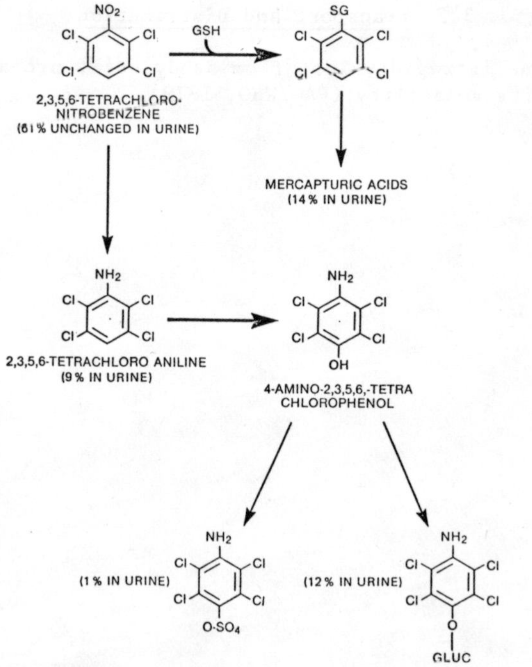

Fig. 1. Tentative biotransformation of tecnazene in rabbits (Adapted from: Betts et al., 1955).

5. STUDIES ON EXPERIMENTAL ANIMALS

5.1 Short-Term Exposures

5.1.1 Single exposure

The acute oral LD_{50} for tecnazene in the rat is 7500 mg/kg body weight (Klimmer, 1971). The acute intraperitoneal LD_{50} in the rat is 3500 mg/kg body weight (Wit et al., 1960).

5.1.2 Repeated exposure

Tecnazene at 0, 1344, or 13 440 mg/kg diet was fed to groups of mice (12 mice per group) for 31 days. No adverse effects were observed at the 1344 mg/kg level, but growth was inhibited at 13 440 mg/kg (Buttle & Dyer, 1950).

Groups of rats (5 males, 5 females per group) received tecnazene at 0, 800, 4000, and 20 000 mg/kg diet for 10 weeks. Death occurred at 20 000 mg/kg; growth was reduced at 4000 mg/kg. There were no effects on growth or mortality rate at 800 mg/kg (Buttle & Dyer, 1950). Tecnazene at 2000 mg/kg, fed to rats for 10 weeks, did not have any effects on the general health, blood picture, autopsy findings, and histological pictures of the liver and kidney. Increased liver and testes weights were observed in the males (no other details reported) (Wit et al., 1960).

Groups of pigs (2 per group) were fed tecnazene at 0, 120, 800, or 1200 mg/kg of potatoes for 26 weeks (1200 mg/kg, equivalent to 7.1 g tecnazene/pig per day or 50 mg/kg body weight). Reduced body weight gains were observed in the first half of the study for the animals in the highest-dose group. General health, and results of haematological tests, and gross and microscopic examination of the liver and kidney were not affected (Abrams et al., 1950).

5.2 Long-Term Exposure

In a 2-year study, groups of beagle dogs (2 males and 2 females per group; controls - 1 male and 1 female) were treated orally (by capsule) with 0, 3.75, 15, 60, or 240 mg tecnazene/kg body weight per day, for 6 days a week. At the 240 mg level, all animals died within the first year of the study, and microscopic changes were observed in liver, kidney, and bone marrow. Growth was normal in all animals at 60 mg/kg, and the clinical chemistry was normal at 15 mg/kg (Donikian et al., unpublished data, 1965).

5.3 Reproduction Studies

In a two-generation reproduction study, groups of rats (5 males and 5 females per group) were fed tecnazene at 0, 200, 800, or 3200 mg/kg diet for 12 weeks, prior to mating. No effects on reproduction were noted at any dose level. Maternal growth was slightly inhibited at the 3200 mg/kg dose level during the 12 week feeding period in each generation, and fatty infiltration of the liver was noted. No effects were observed in the animals on the 800 mg/kg diet (Buttle, unpublished data, 1974).

5.4 Teratogenicity

CD rats and C57B116 mice were administered doses of up to 200 mg tecnazene/kg body weight orally on gestation days 7 - 18. Neither embryotoxic nor teratogenic effects were observed (Courtney et al., 1976). In the same study, CD-1 mice administered the same doses orally on days 7 - 16, also did not show any effects.

5.5 Carcinogenicity

Groups of 65 male and 65 female rats were fed a diet containing tecnazene (purity 99%) at doses of 0, 750, and 1500 mg/kg for 104 weeks. The feeding did not affect general appearance, behaviour, mortality rates, or food consumption. In the second half of the treatment period, a slight reduction in body weight was observed in males in the 1500 mg/kg group. The macropathological findings and non-neoplastic histological changes were those commonly found in the strain used; thus they were not considered to be treatment-related and did not show clear dose relationships. Thirty-nine females of the control group, 48 females of the 750 mg/kg group, and 50 females of the 1500 mg/kg group had benign or malignant tumours of the mammary glands. Adenocarcinomas of the mammary gland were found in 4 females of the control group, 5 in the 750 mg/kg group, and 8 in the 1500 mg/kg group. These differences are of borderline statistical significance (Ben-Dyke et al., unpublished data, 1978a).

Tecnazene (purity 99%) was administered continuously in the diet to 65 male and 65 female mice in each dose group at levels of 0, 750, and 1500 mg/kg for 80 weeks. The only dose-related distribution of neoplasms observed was pulmonary adenoma in the male animals of the 1500 mg/kg group (8 animals showed this lesion, compared with 4 in the control group) (Ben-Dyke et al., unpublished data, 1978b).

6. EFFECTS ON MAN

Occupational dermal sensitivity has been reported in agricultural workers (Lupuknova, 1965).

7. EFFECTS ON THE ENVIRONMENT

Tecnazene has no effect on the bacteria involved in the nitrogen cycle. At 100 mg/kg in a fine sandy loam, no effects were found on the respiration of microorganisms on nitrification (Caseley & Broadbent, 1968).

No other relevant information on the environmental toxicity of tecnazene was found.

8. PREVIOUS EVALUATIONS OF TECNAZENE BY INTERNATIONAL BODIES

The Joint Meeting on Pesticide Residues (JMPR) reviewed residues and toxicity data on tecnazene in 1974, 1978, 1981, and 1983 (FAO/WHO, 1975, 1979, 1982, 1984). Although further toxicological information is still required on tecnazene, the meeting concluded that the no-observed-adverse-effect levels for the rat, mouse, and dog were 750 mg/kg in the diet, 1500 mg/kg in the diet, and 15 mg/kg body weight (by capsule), respectively, and estimated the acceptable daily intake (ADI) for man to be 0 - 0.01 mg/kg body weight.

WHO, in its "Guidelines to the Use of the WHO Recommended Classification of Pesticides by Hazard" (WHO, 1984), classified tecnazene in the list of technical products unlikely to present an acute hazard in normal use.

9. EVALUATION OF HEALTH RISKS FOR MAN AND EFFECTS ON THE ENVIRONMENT

9.1 Evaluation of Health Risks for Man

Tecnazene toxicity

Tecnazene is only slightly toxic according to the scale of Hodge & Sterner (1956). The oral LD_{50} in the rat was 7500 mg/kg body weight. WHO (1978) classified tecnazene in the category of technical products unlikely to present an acute hazard in normal use.

Tecnazene is rapidly absorbed and metabolized in animals after oral administration, and with higher doses, an increasing amount is passed unchanged in the faeces.

In long-term studies the no-observed-adverse-effect levels are:

rat: 750 mg/kg diet, equivalent to 38 mg/kg body weight per day;

mouse: 1500 mg/kg diet, equivalent to 200 mg/kg body weight per day; and

dog: 15 mg/kg body weight per day (administered orally by capsule).

At higher dosage levels tested, growth inhibition occurs and in the dog there are increases in plasma alkaline phosphatase levels.

Tecnazene was neither embryotoxic nor teratogenic in the studies reported. There is no information on mutagenicity or other related short-term tests. Based on the results of an oral feeding study on the mouse and the rat, there are no indications of carcinogenicity.

The only observation in man has been dermal sensitivity.

Exposure to tecnazene

Exposure of the general population is expected to be mainly via residues in food. The residue data available are below the FAO/WHO maximum residue limits.

No data are available on tecnazene levels in air and water and on the levels of occupational exposure.

No cases of human overexposure have been reported.

Hazard assessment

The experimental animal data available indicate that tecnazene (purity greater than 99%) has a low degree of toxicity, even in long-term studies. An acceptable daily intake has been estimated at 0.01 mg/kg body weight.

In the absence of human exposure data, other than residues in food, a factual hazard assessment of present total exposure cannot be made.

The data available on tecnazene would indicate a low degree of concern in relation to human health effects.

9.2 Evaluation of Overall Environmental Effects

In the absence of information on levels in the environment and effects on the environment, such an evaluation cannot be made.

9.3 Conclusions

1. The general population does not seem to be at risk from exposure to tecnazene.

2. With the exception of one report on dermal sensitization in agricultural workers, tecnazene does not seem to be a problem occupationally.

3. With the exception of information on the bacteria involved in the nitrogen cycle there are no available data on other environmental effects. Since the use of this chemical is mainly confined to greenhouses there is little concern for risk to the general environment.

REFERENCES

ABRAMS, T.J., SCORGIE, N.J., & WILLIS, G.A. (1950) Pig feeding trials with 2,3,5,6-tetrachloronitrobenzene. Br. vet. J., 106: 413-420.

BARNES, M.M., JAMES, S.P., & WOOD, P.B. (1959) The formation of mercapturic acids. I. Formation of mercapturic acid and the levels of glutathione in tissues. Biochem. J., 71: 680-690.

BETTS, J.J., JAMES, S.P., & THORPE, W.V. (1955) The metabolism of pentachloronitrobenzene and 2,3,4,6-tetrachloronitrobenzene and the formation of mercapturic acids in the rabbit. Biochem. J., 61: 611-617.

BRAY, H.G., HYBS, Z., JAMES, S.P., & THORPE, W.V. (1953) The metabolism of 2,3,5,6- and 2,3,4,5-tetrachloronitrobenzenes in the rabbit and the reduction of aromatic nitro compounds in the intestine. Biochem. J., 53: 266-273.

BUTTLE, G.A.H. & DYER, F.J. (1950) Experiments on the toxicology of 2,3,5,6-tetrachloronitrobenzene. J. Pharm. Pharmacol., 2: 371-375.

CASELEY, J.C. & BROADBENT, F.E. (1968) The effect of five fungicides on soil respiration and some nitrogen transformations in yolo fine sandy loam. Bull. environ. Contam. Toxicol., 8: 58-64.

COURTNEY, K.D., COPELAND, M.F., & ROBBINS, A. (1976) The effects of pentachloronitrobenzene, hexachlorobenzene and related compounds on fetal development. Toxicol. appl. Pharmacol., 35: 239-256.

DALZIEL, J. & DUNCAN, H.J. (1974) Studies on potato sprout suppressants. I. Residual levels of tecnazene in lab-treated and in commercial samples of potatoes. Potato Res., 17: 215-223.

FAO/WHO (1975) Tecnazene. In: 1974 Evaluations of some pesticide residues in foods, Rome, Food and Agriculture Organization of the United Nations, pp. 531-536.

FAO/WHO (1979) Tecnazene. In: 1978 Evaluations of some pesticide residues in foods, Rome, Food and Agriculture Organization of the United Nations, pp. 227-238.

FAO/WHO (1982) Tecnazene. In: 1981 Evaluations of some pesticide residues in foods, Rome, Food and Agriculture Organization of the United Nations, pp. 43-44.

FAO/WHO (1984) Tecnazene. In: 1983 Evaluations of some pesticide residues in foods, Rome, Food and Agriculture Organization of the United Nations, pp. 44-45.

HODGE, H.C. & STERNER, J.H. (1956) Combined tabulation of toxicity classes. In: Spector, W.S., ed. Handbook of toxicology, Philadelphia, W.B. Saunders Company, Vol. 1.

LUPUKNOVA, K.A. (1965) [Case of occupational toxicodermia caused by 2,3,5,6-tetrachloronitrobenzene.] Gig. Tr. Prof. Zabol., 9: 56-58 (in Russian).

VALANGE, B. (1974) Pesticide residues in fruits and vegetables. Results of a survey performed in 1972. Parasitica, 30: 13-21.

WHO (1984) The WHO recommended classification of pesticides by hazard, Geneva, World health Organization (Unpublished Report VBC/84.2).

WIT, S.L. & REENWANGH, P. (1969) Mercapturic acid formation and enzyme catalyzed conjugations with glutathione in pigeons. Biochem. Biophys. Acta, 177: 329-355.

WIT, S.L., VAN ESCH, G.J., & VAN GENDEREN, H. (1960) Toxicity of some chloronitrobenzene compounds (trichlorodinitrobenzene, trichlorotrinitrobenzene, tetrachloronitrobenzene, and pentachloronitrobenzene) to laboratory rats and residues in food crops treated with these fungicides. In: Proceedings of the 4th International Crop Protection, Hamburg, 1957, Braunschweig, Vol. 2, pp. 1665-1668.

WORTHING, C.R. (1979) The pesticide manual, 6th ed., Croydon, British Crop Protection Council, p. 496.